NOTES
OF
RECENT ADVANCES
IN
CERVICAL INTRAEPITHELIAL
NEOPLASIA

2015
1ST EDITION
DR. PRASAHNT PUJARA

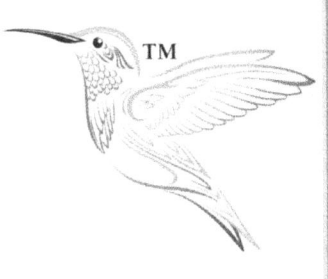

Dedicated to my parents & my bird

PREFACE

This work is the product of study made for final exams for National Board of Examination.

Carcinoma cervix is the leading cancer in women of developing countries & recent updates in the knowledge of it's screening will help caregivers. Proper management of preinvasive lesions of cervix can prevent radical procedures required for invasive lesions of cervix.

The aim is to update the students and clinicians with recent advances in the screening and management of the CERVICAL INTRAEPITHELIAL NEOPLASIA.

I think that I will continue with this series of books for other topics in Obstetrics and Gynecology too in future.

Prashant.

SCREENING OF CERVICAL CANCER

INTRODUCTION

- ACS used detection of **CIN3 as the measure of a screening test's sensitivity for precancer** because **untreated CIN3 has a 30% probability of becoming invasive caner** over a 30 year period, although only about **1% of treated CIN 3 will become invasive.**

- Although CIN2 is the widely accepted threshold for treatment, to provide an additional margin of safety, ACS posited that **CIN2** (which includes some precancer lesions CIN 3 and some lesions CIN 1 that would regress on their own) **should not be the primary target of cervical cancer screening**.

- Screening interval for a particular testing modality should be such that the development of invasive cancer or CIN 3+ is highly unlikely before the next screen.

- Most episodes of HPV infection and many CIN1 and CIN2 cases are transient and will not develop into CIN3 or cancer. Detecting these transient lesions leads to the anxiety associated with a ''positive'' cancer screening test, potential stigmatization from the diagnosis of a sexually transmitted infection, discomfort from additional diagnostic and treatment procedures, bleeding from treatment and longer term, an increased risk of pregnancy complications such as preterm delivery, abortions due to treatment.

- Nearly 100% of cervical cancer cases test positive for HPV.
  - HPV16 is the most carcinogenic HPV genotype and accounts for ~55-60% of all cervical cancers,
  - HPV18 is the next most carcinogenic and accounts for ~10-15% of cervical cancers,
  - Approximately 10 other HPV cause the remaining 25-35% of cervical cancers.

- HPV causes all common and most rare histologic types of cervical cancer. HPV18 causes a greater proportion of glandular cancers, adenocarcinoma and adenosquamous carcinoma than squamous cell carcinoma.

- Sensitivity and specificity of conventional and liquid-based cytology for CIN2+ is same.

- The hallmarks of HPV testing are greater sensitivity but lower specificity for CIN3+ and CIN 2+ and better producibility than cytology.

4 | CIN "screening & management", Dr. Prashant Pujara.

- Reduction in mortality through screening is due to…
  - An increase in the detection of invasive cancer at early stages, when the 5-year survival rate is ~92%,
  - Detection &treatment of preinvasive lesions, which reduces the overall incidence of invasive cancer.

SPECIAL POPULATION

-These guidelines address cervical cancer screening in the general population. These guidelines do not address special, high-risk populations who may need more intensive or alternative screening, e.g., Women
(1) With a history of cervical cancer,
(2) Who were exposed in utero to DES and
(3) Who are immunocompromised (e.g., infection with HIV).

AGE TO BEGIN SCREENING

- Women **less than 21 should not be screened** regardless of age of sexual onset or other risk factors.

- Cervical cancer screening should begin **at age 21**.

RATIONALE

- Cervical cancer is rare in adolescents and young women and may not be prevented by cytology screening.

- Screening adolescents' leads to unnecessary evaluation and potentially to the treatment of preinvasive cervical lesions that have a high probability of regressing spontaneously and that are on average many years fromhaving significant potential for becoming invasive cancer.

- Adolescent cervical cancer prevention should focus on universal HPV vaccination, which is safe, highly efficacious & when used in adolescents before they become sexually active, highly effective & cost-effective.

WOMEN AGED 21-29 YEARS

- Should have a **Pap test every 3 years**. They should not be tested for HPV unless it is needed after an abnormal Pap test result.

- For women aged 21 to29 years with 2 or more consecutive negative cytology results, there is insufficient evidence to support a longer screening interval (i.e., more than 3 years).

RATIONALE

- Rationale for avoiding HPV tests is…
  - Prevalence of carcinogenic HPV approaches 20% in teens & early 20s.
  - Most carcinogenic HPV infections resolve without intervention.
  - Identifying carcinogenic HPV that will resolve leads to repeated call-back, anxiety & interventions without benefit.

WOMEN AGED 30-65 YEARS

- Should be screened with **cytology and HPV testing ("cotesting') every 5 years (preferred)** or cytology alone every 3 years (acceptable).Getting the HPV test with the Pap test at the same time can increase screening intervals up to 5 years for women who do not have HPV & have a normal Pap test result even if they have new sexual partners.)

RATIONALE

- Even with a history of negative cytology tests, the limited evidence **does not support a screening interval longer than 3 years.** Studies report an increased risk of cancer after 3years even after controlling for the prior number of negative cytology tests. Thus 3-year interval for cytology alone provides an appropriate balance.

- The addition of HPV testing to cytology resulted in…
  - Increased detection of prevalent CIN3.
  - Decreased CIN3+ or cancer detection in subsequent screening rounds.
  - Increase in diagnostic lead time with cotesting translates into lower risk following a negative screen, permitting a longer interval between screens with incident cancer rates similar to or lower than screening with cytology alone at shorter intervals.
  - HPV testing provides longer term safety following a negative test than cytology, a useful characteristic for who are screened infrequently.
  - **Enhances the identification of adenocarcinoma of the cervix and its precursors.** Compared with squamous cell cancers, cytology has been relatively ineffective in decreasing the incidence of invasive adenocarcinoma of the cervix.

- The negative predictive value of the HPV test assures women who cotest negative that they are at very low risk for CIN3 and cancer for at least 5 years after negative cotesting.

- The main harms associated with adding HPV testing (the increased referral to colposcopy and diagnosis of CIN 2, some of which would regress without intervention) can be mitigated by extending the screening interval to 5 years and thereby reducing the detection of transient HPV infections and related lesions that would trigger clinical follow-up in low-risk women.

WOMEN AGED OLDER THAN 65 YEARS

- Women **over age 65**with adequate negative prior screening& no history of CIN2+ within the last 20 years should not be screened for cervical cancer.
Adequate negative prior screening is defined as 3 consecutive negative pap smears or2 consecutive negative cotests within 10 years before ceasing screening; with the most recent test occuring within the past 5 years.

- Once screening is discontinued it should not resume for any reason, even if a woman reports having anew sexual partner.

RATIONALE

- CIN2 is rare after age 65.
- HPV risk remains 5-10%.
- Most abnormal screens, even HPV+ are false positive & do not reflect precancer.
- Colposcopy/biopsy/treatment is more difficult.
- Incident HPV infection unlikely to lead to cancer within remaining lifetime.

WOMEN AGED OLDER THAN 65 YEARS WITH A HISTORYOF CIN2, CIN3, OR ADENOCARCINOMA IN SITU

- Following spontaneous regression or appropriate management of CIN2, CIN 3 or AIS, **routine screening should continue for at least 20 years** (even if this extends screening past age 65 years).

RATIONALE

- While women with adequate negative prior screening have a very low risk of cervical cancer, those who have been treated for CIN2+ in the past 20 years (or had it resolve spontaneously) remain at approximately a **5- to 10-foldhigher risk** for cervical cancer than the general population.

- The natural history of incident HPV infections is unaffected by age at acquisition. A new carcinogenic HPV infection in 65 years or older with a cervix should clear spontaneously in most cases, and only a small percentage of women should have a persistent infection. Since the transformation zone of older is smaller and less accessible than in younger , and because cervical cancer develops many years after an incident infection, screening this population would detect a very small number of new cases of CIN2+ and prevent very few cervical cancers and even fewer cancer deaths.

WOMEN WHO HAVE UNDERGONE HYSTERECTOMY & NO HISTORY OF CIN 2+

- Women at any age following a hysterectomy with removal of the cervix who have no history of CIN 2+ **should not be screened for vaginal cancer using any modality.** Evidence of adequate negative prior screening is not required. Once screening is discontinued, it should not resume for any reason, including a woman's report of having a new sexual partner.

RATIONALE

- Vaginal cancer is an uncommon gynecologic malignancy. Its age-specific incidence is similar to or less than that of other cancers for which screening is not performed.

- Women who have had a hysterectomy for cervical intraepithelial lesions may be at an increased risk of vaginal cancer, but the data are limited.

- The incidence rates for all vaginal cancers combined are0.18 per 100,000 female population for in situ cases and0.69 for invasive cases.

- The mean length of time from hysterectomy to an abnormal vaginal cuff cytology result is 19 years.

- Even if women with hysterectomy are at an increased risk of vaginal cancer, there is **no proven method to effectively intervene before vaginal cancer develops**.

SCREENING FOLLOWING VACCINATION

- Women who have had the HPV vaccine should still follow the screening recommendations for their age group.

RATIONALE

- HPV16/18 vaccination is highly effective in preventing CIN2 and CIN3 among women not previously exposed to these types of HPV.

- Vaccinating women up to age 26 years, many women may be vaccinated after HPV infection has already occurred, when efficacy declines.

- At low coverage, herd immunity will not occur, and there will be little impact on HPV transmission rates and consequently on the incidence of CIN3+.

- Current screening recommendations may be modified following HPV vaccination; which will take more than a decade to see the full impact of vaccination on screening outcomes.

- Vaccination is expected to reduce the prevalence of high-grade cervical lesions over time, which will have a deleterious influence on the positive predictive value of screening tests, thus increasing the proportion of false-positive results.

- Many questions are still unanswered...
- The duration of protection following HPV vaccination, especially in girls aged 11 years to 12 years, and the impact on age-specific cancer risks.
- Reliable documentation of fully vaccinated status at an age likely to be prior to HPV exposure would be needed.
- The effect of vaccination on the HPV genotype distribution.
- The impact of vaccination on the performance of cytology and HPV testing.
- The effect of vaccination on screening adherence.

SCREENING WITH HPV TESTING ALONE

- Women aged 30 years to 65 years should not be screened with HPV testing alone as an alternative to cotesting at 5-year intervals or cytology alone at 3-year intervals.

RATIONALE& EVIDENCE

- HPV testing has increased sensitivity for the detection of CIN3+ and CIN2+ after a single screening round. Greater sensitivity also means greater negative predictive value over a longer time period, because the absence of positive HPV findings is an indication of a low risk of developingCIN3+. RCTs have been **less successful at defining the specificity of HPV testing,** and therefore the potential harms of primary HPV testing are poorly quantified.

- HPV testing is more sensitive for the detection of CIN2+ & CIN3+ than cytology alone and is almost as sensitive as cotesting. In addition, a negative HPV test provides greater reassurance against CIN3+ in the subsequent 5 to 7 years than cytology alone and is nearly as reassuring as a negative cotest. Therefore an acceptable screening interval for the use of HPV testing alone should be comparable to that of cotesting.

- The published studies of HPV testing alone for primary screening are limited by a lack of long-term follow-up, HPV testing alone for primary screening is less specific than cytology alone and may identify clinically insignificant disease that is destined to spontaneously regress. Thus, a strategy of immediate colposcopy of all HPV-positive women can be associated with significant harms due to unnecessary diagnostic procedures or treatment, which may outweigh the benefits of the increased sensitivity.

- Other strategies have aimed to improve specificity and reduce harm by interposing secondary testing for management decisions between a positive HPV test and colposcopy. Potential secondary biomarkers included **HPV genotyping (for HPV16 or HPV16/18), HPV mRNA testing, and/or the detection of other non-HPV biomarkers (e.g., p16INK4A).**

- The **lack of a well-defined and evaluated management strategy** for positive tests precludes their practical implementation.

- The **lack of an internal standard for specimen adequacy for some HPV assays** may provide false reassurance among a small number of women whose negative screening results may be a function of specimen inadequacy rather than the true absence of disease. Such an event is less common with cytology since specimen adequacy assessment is a routine component of the evaluation, and inadequacy prompts intervention and follow-up on the part of the clinician and patient. Thus, the inclusion of cytology with HPV testing (i.e., cotesting) provides some additional reassurance against testing errors due to specimen inadequacy, although the benefits in terms of sensitivity and negative predictive values are only incremental.

MANAGEMENT OF ABNORMAL SCREENING TESTS

INTRODUCTION

- Women aged 30-64 years with a negative co-test have a 5 year risk of CIN3+ of only 8/10,000.

- Role of endocervical sampling is controversial. Indications are ASC-US, LSIL, ASC-H & HSIL. Endocervical brushing has better sensitivity than curettage with similar specificity, better tolerance & fewer insufficient samples, although grading may be more difficult because stroma is rarely sampled with brushing. Either is acceptable for endocervical sampling.

- Both ablation and excision effectively treat CIN.

- Margin status is convenient predictor of recurrence and a traditional risk marker, although not an independent risk factor.

- HPV testing is more sensitive but less specific than cytology in post treatment follow up of CIN & it may result in earlier diagnosis of persistent or recurrent disease.

- In 2011, women of 30-64 years, followed after positive HPV tests but negative cytology were referred to colposcopy only if they had LSIL or more severe cytology or a positive HPV test during surveillance co-testing. However, only 0.04% of all women aged 30-64 years in the database had HPV negative ASC-US after an HPV-positive, cytology negative result, so referring them for colposcopy will burden care systems minimally. Thus, **colposcopy is recommended for any positive HPV test or any abnormal cytology during follow-up.**

- Immunosuppressed with abnormal results should be managed in the same manner as immunocompetent.

UNSATISFACTORY CYTOLOGY

- Incidence is 1% or less.
- Unreliable for detecting epithelial abnormalities.
- Causes are…
  - Blood, inflammation or other processes (in conventional cytology) &
  - Insufficient squamous cells (in liquid based media).

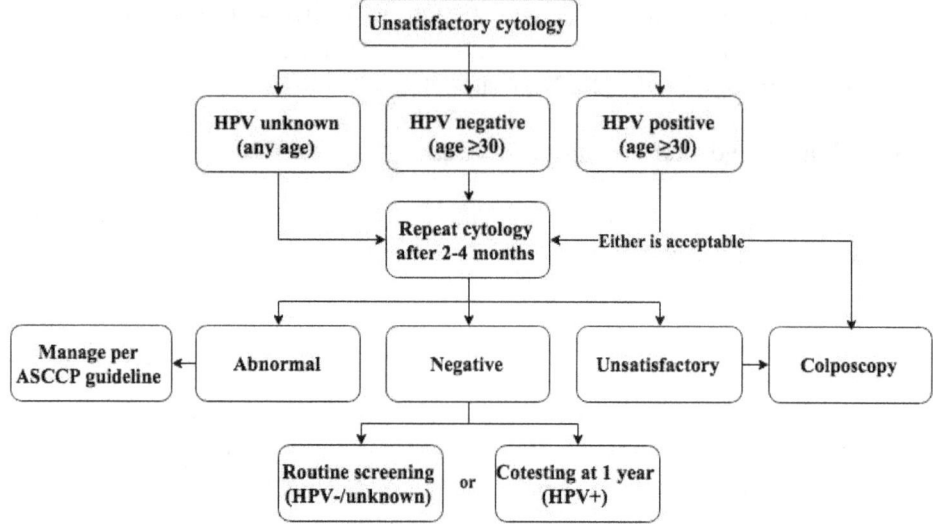

NEGATIVE CYTOLOGY BUT ABSENT OR INSUFFICIENT EC/TZ COMPONENT

- Incidence is 10-20% and higher in older women.
- Has adequate cellularity for interpretation but lacks endocervical or metaplastic cells, suggesting that the squamocolumnar junction may not have been adequately sampled.
- Raises concern for missed disease.
- However, they have fewer concurrent cytologic abnormalities; they don't have a higher risk for CIN3+ over time than women with satisfactory EC/TZ component. The lower rate of cytologic abnormality appears to occur because women whose cytology lacks a satisfactory EC/TZ are older, and older women have lower CIN+ risk.
- Negative cytology has good specificity and negative predictive value despite absent or insufficient EC/TZ.
- An absent EC/TZ is not associated with an increased incidence of cervical disease after treatment of CIN2+.

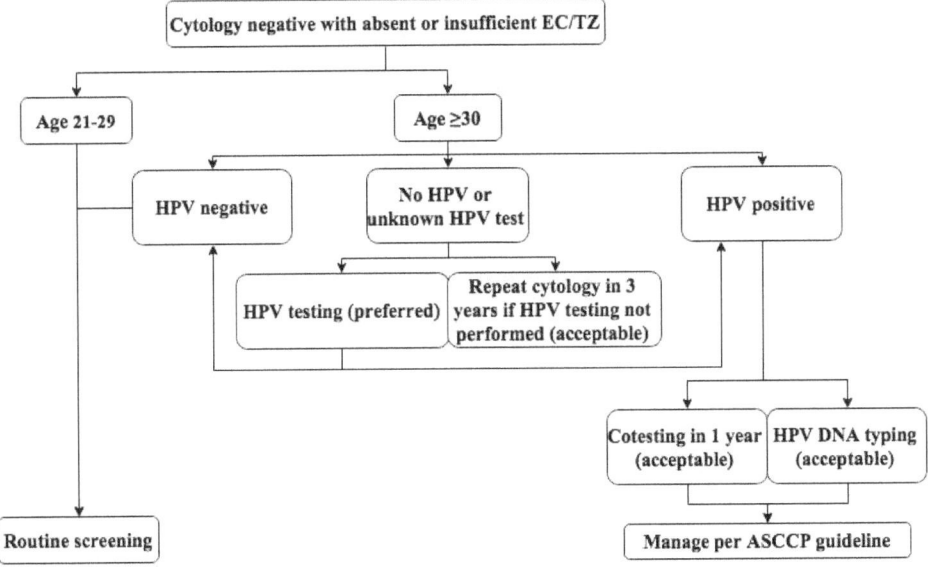

- If HPV type 16 or type 18 is present on HPV DNA typing, colposcopy is recommended. If HPV type 16 and type 18 are absent, repeat co-testing in 12 >months is recommended.

NEGATIVE CYTOLOGY WITH POSITIVE HPV TEST

- They are at higher risk for later CIN3+ than negative HPV test.

- The CIN3+ risk for every co-test result obtained after an initial HPV positive but cytology negative result is higher than risk associated with that co-test result in women with prior negative screening.

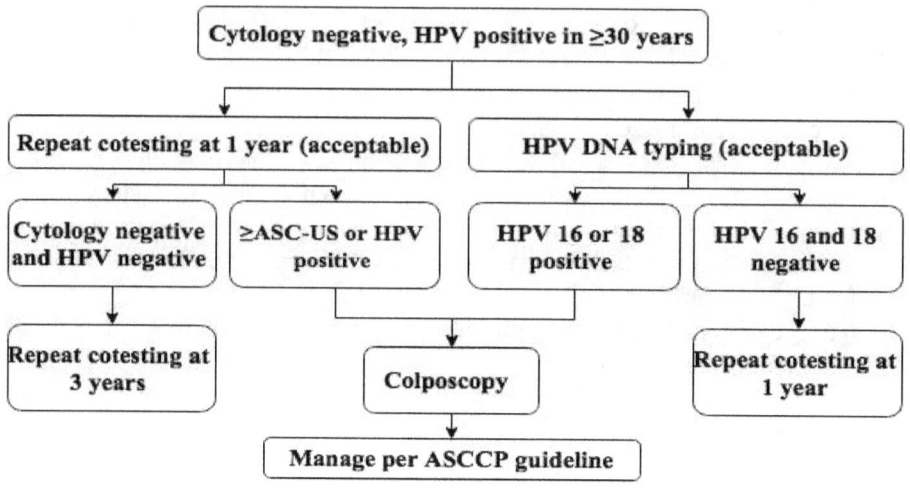

ASC-US

- MC cytologic abnormality.

- The lowest risk of CIN3+, partly because $1/3^{rd}$ to $2/3^{rd}$ are not HPV associated.

- Though the absolute risk of CIN3+ is low after HPV negative ASC-US, it is comparable to CIN3+ risk among women with negative cytology alone than those with a negative co-test, suggesting a 3 year interval for follow-up.

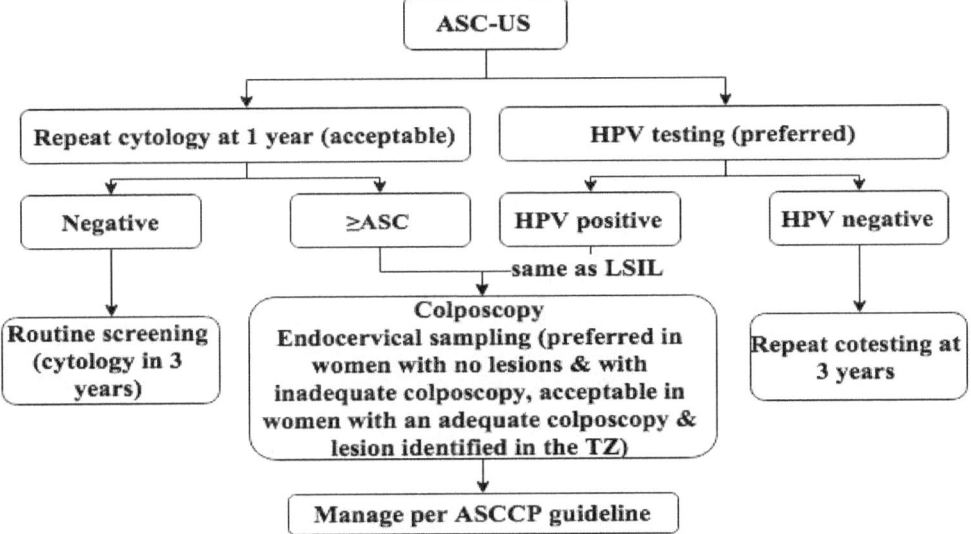

- When colposcopy doesn't identify CIN in HPV positive ASC-US, co-testing at 12 months is recommended. If the co-test is HPV negative & cytology negative, return for age appropriate testing in 3 years is recommended. If all tests are negative at that time, routine screening is recommended.

- HPV testing in follow-up after colposcopy should not be performed at intervals of less than 12 months.

- HPV negative and ASC-US...
  - Should be followed with co-testing at 3 years rather than 5 years and
  - Are insufficient to allow exit from screening at age 65 years.

ASC-US in special populations

Women 21-24 years

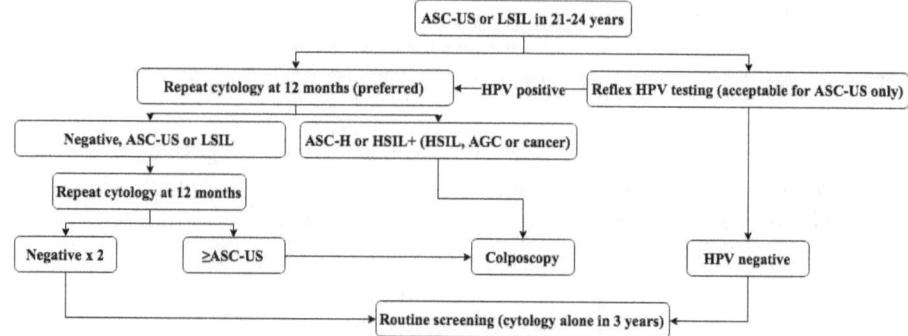

Pregnant

- Identical to nonpregnant, with the exception that deferring colposcopy until 6 weeks postpartum is acceptable.
- Endocervical curettage is unacceptable.
- Who have no cytologic, histologic or colposcopically suspected CIN2+ at the initial colposcopy, postpartum follow up is recommended.

Women ≥ 65 years or postmenopausal

- Same as general population, except when considering exit from screening for ≥ 65 years.
- For those, HPV negative ASC-US results should be considered abnormal.
- Additional surveillance is recommended with repeat screening in 1 year; co-testing is preferred but cytology is acceptable.

LSIL

- Natural history of LSIL approximates that of HPV positive ASC-US, suggesting that either should be managed similarly.
- LSIL in 20-24 years carries a lower risk of CIN3+ than older.
- LSIL is highly associated with HPV infection.
- The risk of CIN3+ in HPV negative with LSIL is low similar to that of ASC-US alone.

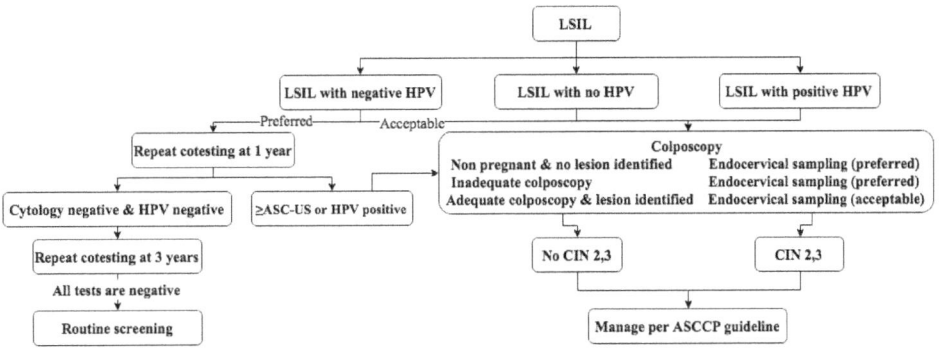

LSIL in special populations

Women 21-24 years (same as ASC-US in 21-24 years)

Pregnant

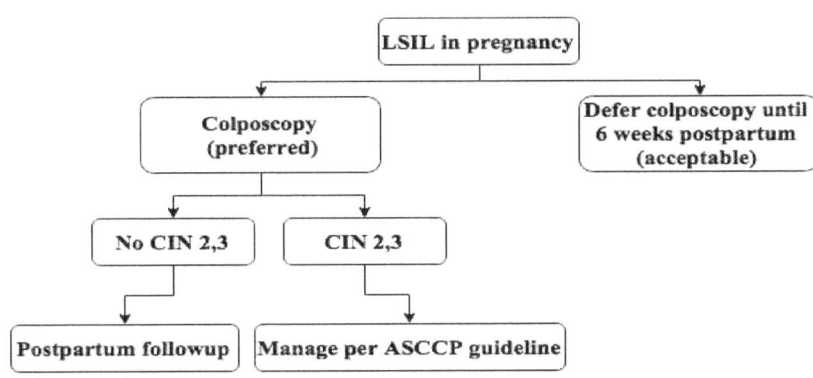

- Endocervical curettage is unacceptable.
- For pregnant women aged 21-24 years, follow-up according to the guidelines for management of LSIL in women aged 21-24 years is recommended.

Postmenopausal

- Acceptable options in postmenopausal with LSIL & no HPV test include…
  - HPV testing,
  - Repeat cytological testing at 6 months and 12 months,
  - Colposcopy.

- If the HPV test is negative or if CIN is not identified at colposcopy, repeat cytology in 12 months is recommended.

- If either the HPV test is positive or repeat cytology is ASC-US or greater, colposcopy is recommended.

- If two consecutive repeat cytology tests are negative, return to routine screening is recommended.

ASC-H

- ASC-H confers higher risk for CIN3+ over time than ASC-US or LSIL, although risk is lower than following HSIL.

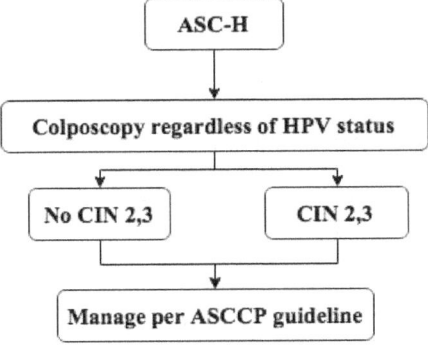

ASC-H in special populations

Women 21-24 years

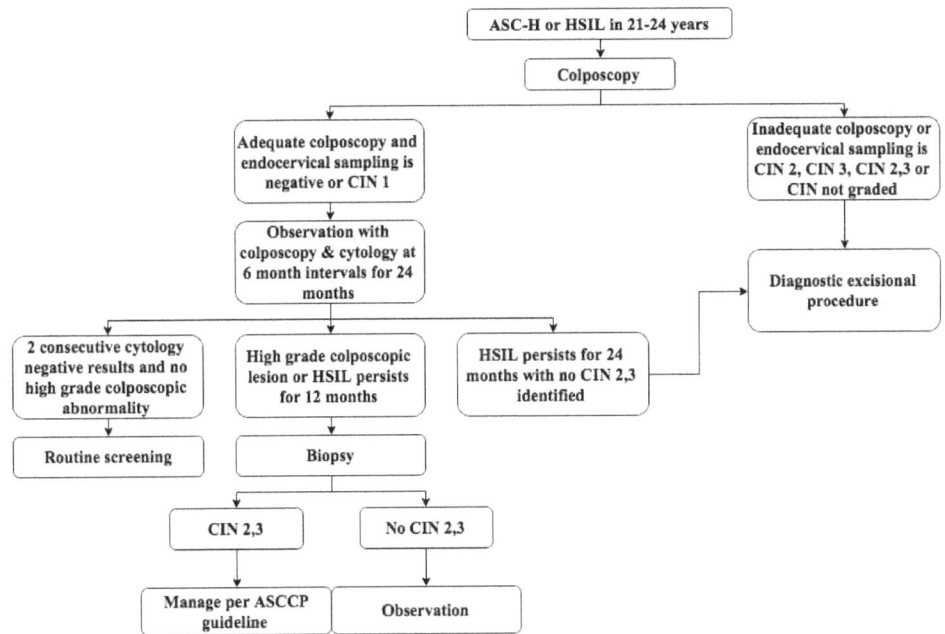

HSIL

- CIN2+ is found at colposcopy in ~60% of HSIL. This justifies immediate excision of the transformation zone, especially those who are at risk for loss to follow-up or who have completed childbearing.

- Cervical cancer is found at colposcopy in ~2% of HSIL, although risk rises with age and is low among aged 21-24 years, even with follow-up.

- Five-year cervical cancer risk is 8% among women 30 years of age and older.

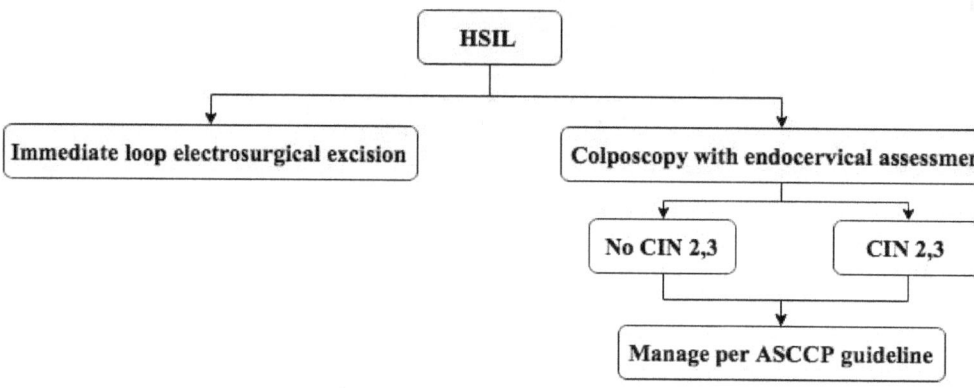

- A diagnostic excisional procedure is recommended in HSIL when the colposcopic examination is inadequate, except during pregnancy.

- Ablation is unacceptable when…
  - Colposcopy has not been performed,
  - CIN 2,3 is not identified histologically,
  - Endocervical assessment identifies CIN 2, CIN 3, CIN 2,3 or ungraded CIN.

HSIL in special populations

Women 21-24 years (same as ASC-H in 21-24 years)

AGC, AIS & BENIGN GLANDULAR CHANGES

- AGC…
  - Interpretation is poorly reproducible and uncommon,
  - Has been associated with polyps and metaplasia but also with neoplasias, including adenocarcinomas of the endometrium, cervix, ovary, fallopian tube and other sites,
  - Is most commonly associated with squamous lesions including CIN 1.

- Neoplasia risk is higher when reported as AGC favor neoplasia or frank AIS.

- Although cervical adenocarcinoma is HPV associated and can be detected with HPV testing, endometrial cancer is not, so reflex HPV testing does not identify a subgroup that need less invasive assessment. A negative HPV test can be useful in identifying women at greater risk for endometrial rather than cervical disease.

-Benign-appearing endometrial cells and stromal cells or histiocytesin post-menopausal women can be associated with ~5% risk of clinically important pathology including endometrial adenocarcinoma,

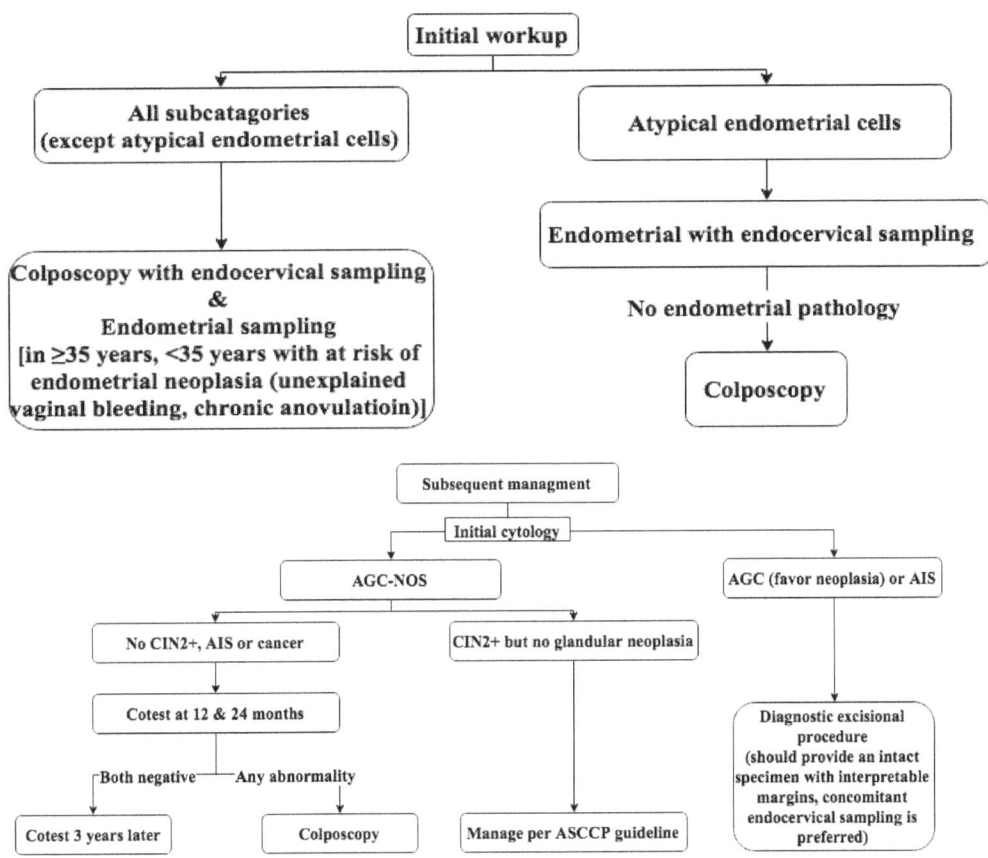

AGC or AIS in special populations

Women 21-24 years (same for all)

Pregnant (Identical to nonpregnant, except that endocervical curettage and endometrial biopsy are unacceptable)

Benign glandular changes

- For...
- Asymptomatic premenopausal women, no further evaluation is recommended,
- Postmenopausal women, endometrial assessment is recommended,
- Post-hysterectomy patients, no further evaluation is recommended.

CIN 1 AND NO CIN FOUND AT COLPOSCOPY AFTER ABNORMAL CYTOLOGY

- CIN 1 is the histologic manifestation of HPV infection.

- Although most CIN 1 lesions are associated with oncogenic HPV, nononcogenic HPV types are also commonly found.

- The natural history of CIN1issimilartothatofHPV-positiveASC-USandLSIL in the absence of CIN.

- Regression rates are high in younger, andprogressiontoCIN2+is uncommon.

- TheriskofoccultCIN3+withCIN1at colposcopic biopsy is linked to the risk conveyed by prior cytology (low risk in ASC-US or LSIL, but high risk after HSIL, ASC-H, and AGC).

- Failure to detect CIN 2+ at colposcopy in women with HSIL does not mean that a CIN 2+ lesion has been excluded, although occult carcinoma is unlikely. As a result, women with HSIL who do not have immediate diagnostic excision require close follow-up.

- Since CIN 3+ risk is elevated with either HPV-16 or HPV-18 or persistent oncogenic HPV infection of any type even when cytology is negative, guidelines must provide for follow-up for women with these ''lesser abnormalities'' even when no CIN is found. These **''lesser abnormalities'' include HPV-16 or HPV-18 positivity, persistent untyped oncogenic HPV, ASC-US, and LSIL.**

- Current guidelines on management of CIN 1 on endocervical sampling do not apply when CIN 2, CIN 3, or CIN 2,3 is specified or when the lesion seen cannot be graded, as an associated invasive cancer cannot be excluded without a diagnostic excision procedure.

- Hysterectomy as the primary and principal treatment for histologically diagnosed CIN 1 is unacceptable.

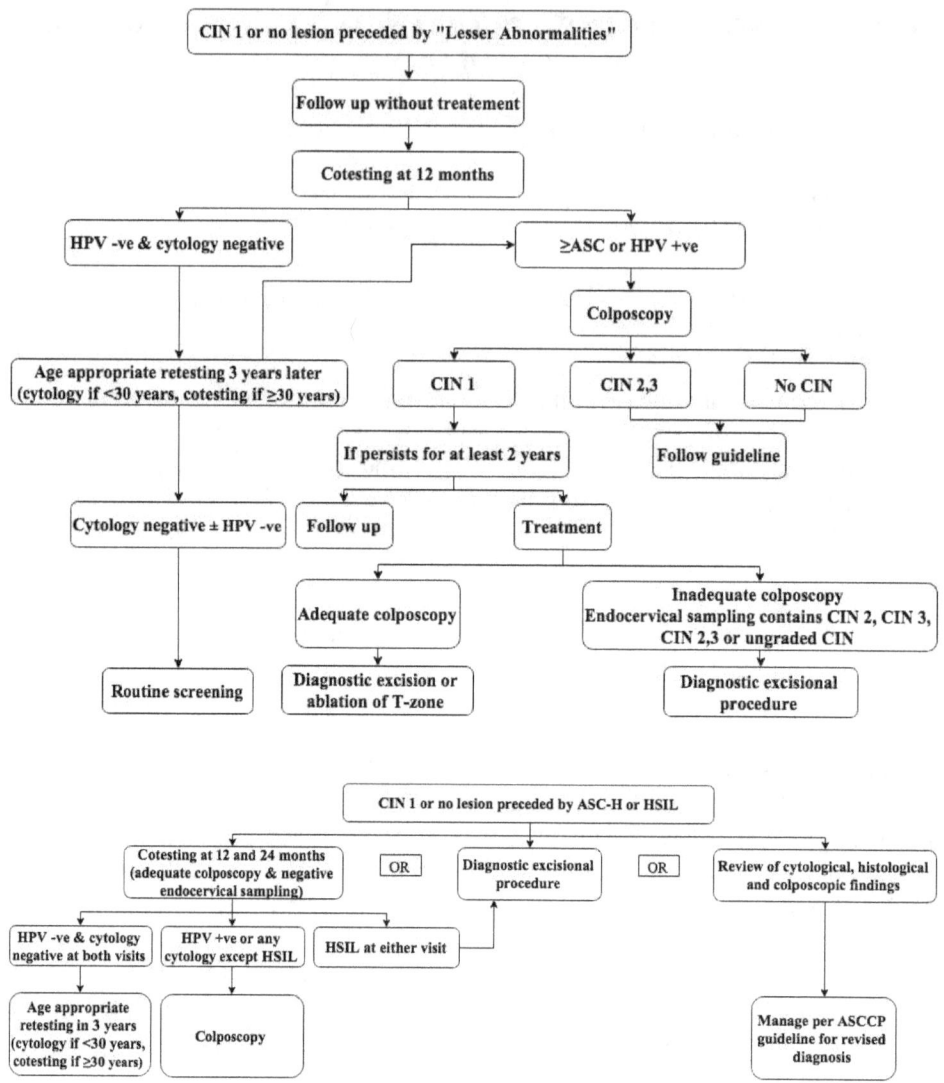

CIN 1 on endocervical sampling

- When CIN 1 is detected on endocervical sampling after...
  - Lesser abnormalities on cytology but no CIN 2+ is detected in colposcopic biopsies, follow ASCCP management guidelines for CIN 1, with the addition of repeat endocervical sampling in 12 months.
  - ASC-H, HSIL, or AGC on cytology or with a colposcopic biopsy reported as CIN 2+, management according to specific abnormality is recommended.

For women not treated, repeat endocervical sampling at the time of evaluation for the other abnormality is recommended.

CIN 1 in special populations

Women 21-24 years

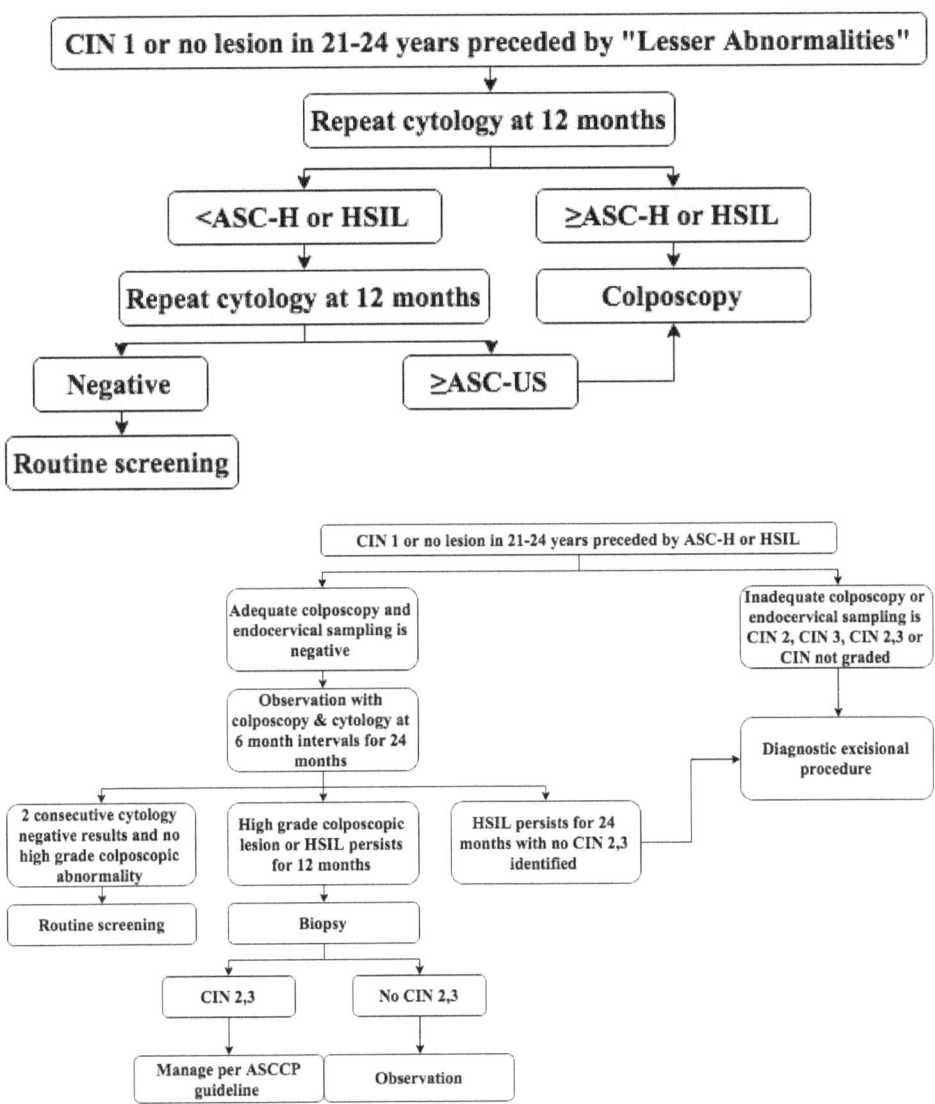

- Regardless of antecedent cytolgoy, treatment of CIN 1 in 21-24 years is not recommended.

Pregnant

- Follow-up without treatment is recommended. Treatment of pregnant for CIN 1 is unacceptable.

CIN 2, CIN 3 AND CIN 2,3

- CIN 2 remains the consensus threshold for treatment.

- Confirmed CIN 3 is the immediate precursor to invasive cancer and should not be observed, regardless of age or concern about future fertility.

- Hysterectomy is unacceptable as primary therapy for CIN 2, CIN 3 or CIN 2,3.

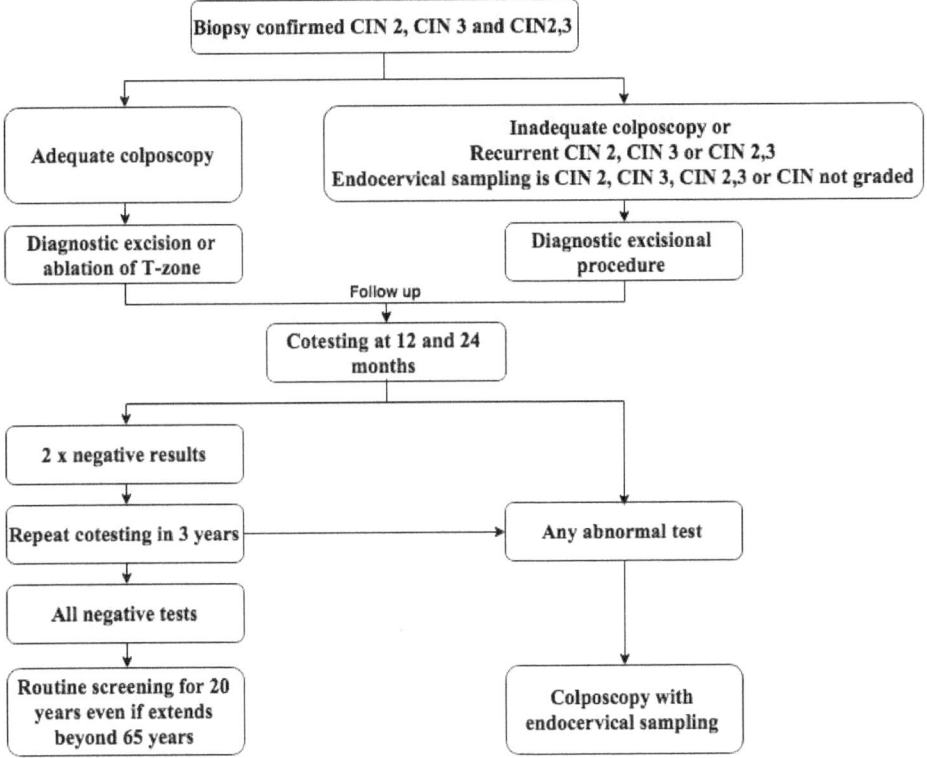

- Repeat treatment or hysterectomy based on a positive HPV test is unacceptable.

- If CIN 2, CIN 3, or CIN 2,3 is identified at the margins of a diagnostic excisional procedure or in an endocervical sample obtained immediately after the treatment…
   - Reassessment using cytology with endocervical sampling at 4-6months (preferred),
   - Repeat diagnostic excisional procedure (acceptable),
   - Hysterectomy if a repeat diagnostic procedure is not feasible (acceptable).

- A repeat diagnostic excisional procedure or hysterectomy is acceptable for recurrent or persistent CIN 2, CIN 3 or CIN 2,3.

CIN 2, CIN 2 or CIN 2,3 in special populations

Women 21-24 years

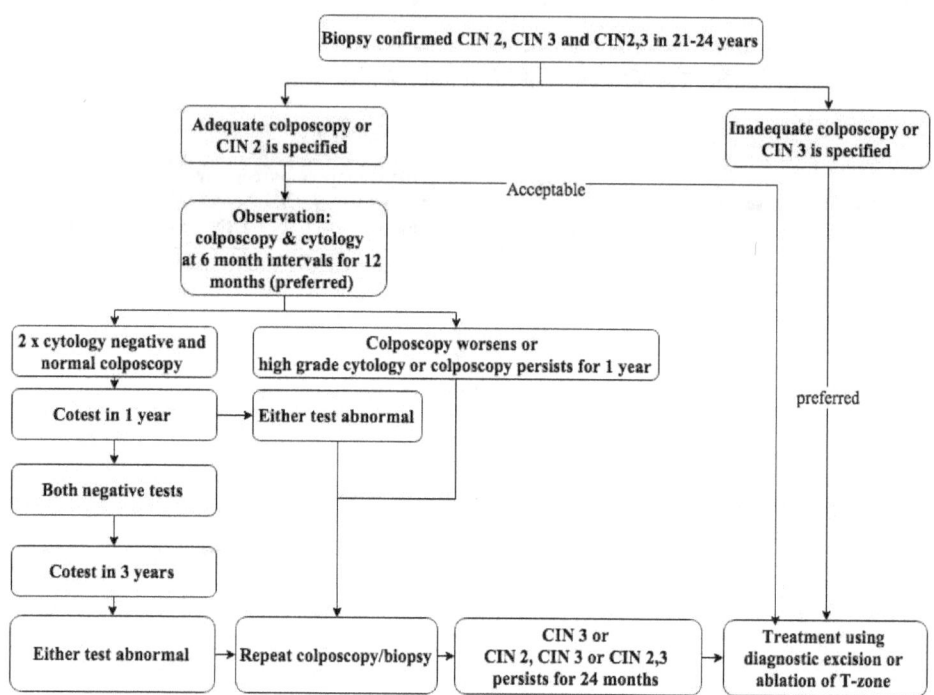

- Follow up according to guidelines for treated CIN 2, CIN 3 or CIN 2,3 is recommended.

Pregnant

- In the absence of invasive disease or advanced pregnancy, additional colposcopic and cytologic examinations are acceptable at intervals of every 12 weeks.
- Repeat biopsy only if the appearance of the lesion worsens or if cytology suggests invasive cancer.
- A diagnostic excisional procedure is recommended only if invasion is suspected. Unless invasive cancer is identified, treatment is unacceptable.
- Deferring re-evaluation with cytology and colposcopy until at least 6 weeks postpartum is acceptable.

AIS

- The incidence of AIS is low but rising.

- Colposcopic changes associated with AIS can be minimal, so determining the limits of a lesion can be difficult.

- AIS frequently extend into the endocervical canal, complicating determination of the desired depth of excision.

- AIS can be multifocal and discontinuous, so negative margins on an excision specimen do not provide assurance that the disease has been completely excised.

- Diagnostic excision is allowed using any modality, but specimen should be intact and margins should be interpretable, avoid fragmentation of the specimen, including ''top-hat'' serial endocervical excisions. This may require use of larger loops than those employed to excise visible squamous lesions.

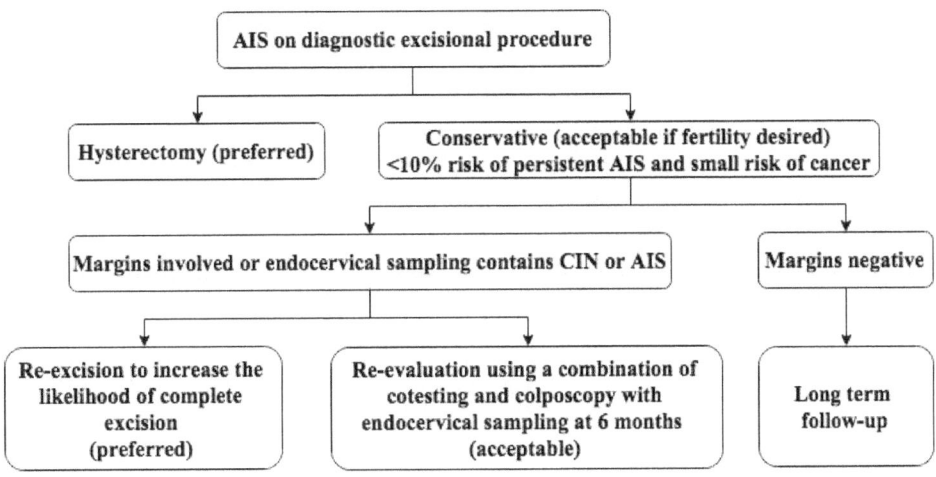

IMPORTANT TERMINOLOGY

- **Adequate colposcopy** indicates that the entire squamocolumnar junction and the margins of any visible lesion can be visualized with the colposcope.

- **Co-testing** is assessment for cervical disease using a combination of cytology and HPV testing at the same time, regardless of the cytology result.

- **Reflex HPV testing** is the performance of HPV testing only in response to an abnormality to stratify risk and guide further management.

- **Endometrial sampling** includes obtaining a specimen for histologic evaluation using an endometrial biopsy, dilation and curettage, or hysteroscopy.

- **Endocervical sampling** includes obtaining a specimen for either histologic evaluation using an endocervical curette or a cytobrush or for cytologic evaluation using a cytobrush.

- **Endocervical assessment** is the process of evaluating the endocervical canal for the presence of neoplasia using either a colposcope or endocervical sampling.

- **Diagnostic excisional procedure** is the process of obtaining a specimen from the transformation zone and endocervical canal for histologic evaluation and includes laser conization, cold-knife conization, loop or needle electrosurgical excision, and loop electrosurgical conization.

- CIN 3+ (CIN 3, AIS and cancer) & CIN 2+ (CIN 2 and CIN 3+).

- Histopathology results reported as LSIL should be managed as CIN 1 and those reported as HSIL should be managed as CIN 2,3.

www.ingramcontent.com/pod-product-compliance
Lightning Source LLC
Chambersburg PA
CBHW070757180526
45168CB00004B/1645